Swing Strong: Golfing Fitness For Seniors

by D. Patrick

SWING STRONG: GOLFING FITNESS FOR SENIORS

D. PATRICK

Mookango Publishing

This book is not intended as a substitute for consultation with a licensed healthcare practitioner, such as your doctor. Before you begin any healthcare/exercise program, or change your lifestyle in any way, you should consult your physician or another medical professional to ensure that you are in good health and that the examples contained in this book will not harm you.

Chapter 1: Welcome to Swing Strong: Golfing Fitness For Seniors

As you embark on your golfing journey in your golden years, it's important to recognize the unique needs and considerations of senior golfers. Golf is a sport that can be enjoyed at any age, but it's crucial to ensure you're taking care of your body and optimizing your physical fitness to enhance your game and prevent injury.

Swing Strong is here to guide you on this path. This guide is designed specifically for senior golfers who wish to improve their overall fitness and performance on the course. Whether you're a seasoned golfer or just starting out, we understand that every golfer is unique and may face different challenges as they age. Through tailored exercises and techniques, we will provide you with the knowledge and tools to navigate these challenges and take your golf game to the next level.

So, why focus on fitness for senior golfers? The truth is, as we age, our bodies undergo various changes that can impact our ability to move, swing, and perform at our best. Loss of muscle mass, reduced flexibility, and decreased stamina are common physical changes experienced by seniors. These factors can affect your swing mechanics, power, and overall performance on the course. However, with a well-rounded fitness program, specially designed for senior golfers, you can combat these age-related factors and maintain your strength, flexibility, and endurance to continue enjoying the sport you love.

The benefits of fitness for senior golfers extend far beyond the golf course. Regular exercise not only improves your golf game but also has a positive impact on your overall health and well-being. Engaging in physical activity helps to maintain a healthy weight, reduce the risk of chronic diseases such as heart disease and diabetes, and improve bone density. It also enhances cognitive function, promotes mental clarity, and reduces stress and anxiety.

Throughout this book, we will cover a wide range of topics related to golfing fitness for seniors. We will explore the benefits of fitness for senior golfers in more detail, emphasizing the positive impact it has on your game and overall quality of life.

Let's start by delving deeper into the importance of flexibility for senior golfers. As we age, our muscles and connective tissues naturally become less supple, leading to reduced flexibility. This can affect your golf swing by limiting your ability to rotate your torso and shoulders fully. Consequently, you may experience a shorter backswing and reduced clubhead speed. To counteract this, we will guide you through a variety of stretching exercises that target key areas of your body, such as the shoulders, hips, and hamstrings. These stretches will help improve your range of motion, allowing you to achieve a full and unrestricted backswing, resulting in a more fluid and consistent swing.

Next, let's explore the importance of strength training for senior golfers. Building strength in specific muscle groups used in the golf swing can lead to improved power, stability, and control. Strengthening your core muscles, which include the abdominals, hip muscles, and lower back muscles, is essential for a stable and powerful golf swing foundation. Additionally, exercises targeting the shoulders, forearms, and legs will support a more controlled and efficient swing. By engaging in a regular strength training routine, you'll be able to generate more power, maintain consistency, and reduce the risk of injury.

Maintaining balance is another crucial aspect for senior golfers. As we age, our balance can deteriorate, increasing the risk of falls and affecting our stability during the swing. Balance exercises will not only improve your performance on the golf course but also enhance your overall mobility and reduce the risk of injuries in daily life. We will provide exercises and drills aimed at improving your balance and stability, ensuring you maintain a strong and cantered posture throughout your swing. These exercises can be done both on and off the golf course to reinforce your stability in all aspects of life.

Endurance is another vital element of golfing fitness for seniors. A round of golf can be physically demanding, requiring stamina and energy. Engaging in regular cardiovascular exercise, such as walking, swimming, or cycling, will improve your cardiovascular fitness, enabling you to play 18 holes with less fatigue. Additionally, targeted endurance exercises, such as interval training and circuit workouts, can condition your body for the demands of the golf course, allowing you to maintain focus and performance throughout your round.

While physical fitness is crucial, we must not overlook the mental aspect of golfing. Cultivating focus, resilience, and a positive mindset can greatly impact your overall performance on the course. We will provide strategies and tips to help you stay mentally sharp and bounce back from setbacks, enabling you to stay in the game and maintain your confidence throughout your round. Techniques such as visualization, mindfulness, and positive self-talk can enhance your mental game and allow you to perform at your best under pressure.

Lastly, we will discuss injury prevention and recovery strategies to ensure you're taking care of your body and minimizing the risk of setbacks. We will delve into common golf-related injuries, such as golfers elbow, lower back pain, and rotator cuff issues, and provide guidance on injury prevention exercises, warm-up routines, and proper technique to protect your body and keep you playing the game you love for years to come. By being proactive about injury prevention and recovery, you can continue to enjoy golf without being hindered by pain or discomfort.

Through a combination of expert advice, exercise demonstrations, and practical tips, Swing Strong strives to empower senior golfers to optimize their physical fitness and elevate their game. Whether you're looking to improve your swing mechanics, increase your distance off the tee, or simply enjoy the game with reduced risk of injury, this book is your comprehensive guide to achieving those goals.

So, grab your clubs, put on your golf shoes, and get ready to embark on a transformative journey of golfing fitness. Let's swing strong and make the most out of every round on the golf course!

Chapter 2: Embracing Your Golfing Journey in Your Golden Years

As we enter our golden years, it's essential to recognize that age is just a number when it comes to pursuing our passions. Golf, a sport beloved by many, is no exception. In fact, fo seniors, it can be a wonderful opportunity to stay active, socialize, and continue challenging oneself.

Embracing your golfing journey in your golden years begins with a positive mindset. It's crucial to approach the game with enthusiasm, embracing the joy it brings rather than focusing on limitations. Understand that your golfing abilities may change with age, but that doesn't mean you can't still experience growth and enjoyment on the course.

One of the most significant advantages of golf for seniors is the opportunity to spend time outdoors. Being surrounded by nature, breathing in the fresh air, and enjoying the beauty of the golf course can have a profound impact on your overall well-being. It's a chance to connect with nature and find solace from the stresses of everyday life.

Furthermore, golf is a social sport, providing ample opportunities for interaction and friendship. Whether you join a senior golf league, participate in tournaments, or simply play a round with friends, you'll have the chance to bond with fellow golfers who share your love for the game. Building and maintaining connections through golf can enrich your social life and contribute to a sense of belonging and fulfilment.

It's essential to acknowledge that golf can also bring challenges as we age. Physical limitations may arise, and certain aspects of the game may require adjustments. However, embracing these challenges and finding ways to overcome them is part of the journey. Adapting your approach to the game can make it more enjoyable and sustainable in the long run. As a senior golfer, it's beneficial to prioritize flexibility and mobility exercises to maintain and improve your range of motion. Stretching before and after rounds can help loosen muscles and prevent injuries. Learning proper techniques, such as using modified swings or equipment tailored to your needs, can also make the game more accessible and comfortable. Consider seeking out resources that cater specifically to senior golfers, such as instructional videos or lessons tailored to address the nuances of playing golf as you age. Learning from experienced professionals who understand the unique needs of senior golfers can significantly enhance your experience on the course.

Maintaining a healthy lifestyle is another crucial aspect of embracing your golfing journey as a senior. Engaging in regular exercise, such as walking or cycling, can improve cardiovascular health, strength, and stamina. Strengthening core muscles through exercises like yoga or Pilates can also contribute to a more stable and balanced swing. Additionally, practicing mindfulness and stress-reduction techniques can help you stay present and focused during your rounds. Eating a balanced diet, staying hydrated, and getting enough sleep are also vital components of maintaining optimal performance on the course. By taking care of your body and mind, you'll have the energy, stamina, and mental clarity needed to excel in your golfing endeavours.

Moreover, golfing in your golden years offers a unique opportunity for personal growth and self-reflection. The game requires focus, patience, and perseverance—qualities that can be honed on the course and carried into other areas of your life. Through golf, you'll learn to embrace challenges, develop problem-solving skills, and cultivate resilience. The process of improving your golf game can be a metaphor for the journey of life, teaching you valuable lessons about dedication, adaptability, and the importance of enjoying the moment. As you navigate the greens and fairways, take the time to appreciate the little things—the chirping birds, the gentle breeze, and the camaraderie shared with fellow golfers. Celebrate the beauty of the game itself, the crisp sound of a well-struck ball, and the satisfaction of seeing it land where you intended. Embrace the inevitable ups and downs and find solace in the journey rather than solely focusing on the destination.

Remember, your golfing journey is deeply personal. It's not about comparing yourself to others or trying to achieve unrealistic expectations. Golf is a game that can be enjoyed at any skill level, and the real value lies in the process and the experiences it brings.

So, embrace your golfing journey in your golden years. Stay positive, stay active, and savour every moment you spend on the course. It's a remarkable opportunity to continue growing, learning, and connecting with both yourself and others. Remember, age is no barrier to the joys of golf. Enjoy the process, take care of your body and mind, and let the magic of the game unfold as you navigate the beautiful greens and fairways of life.

Chapter 3: The Benefits of Fitness for Senior Golfers

As we age, staying physically active becomes increasingly important for maintaining our overall health and well-being. When it comes to golf, staying fit and incorporating exercise into our routine can have numerous benefits for senior golfers. In this chapter, we will explore the many advantages that fitness can bring to your golf game as a senior.

First and foremost, regular exercise can improve your physical fitness by increasing your strength, flexibility, and cardiovascular endurance. These three components are essential for a strong and effective golf swing. By engaging in strength training exercises, such as resistance training or weightlifting, you can target specific muscles used in the golf swing, such as the core, legs, and shoulders, which will help generate more power and stability in your shots. Strengthening the core muscles is particularly important, as it provides a solid foundation for a consistent and controlled swing. A stronger body will also help prevent injuries and enable you to maintain proper posture and alignment throughout your swing, reducing the risk of strain or discomfort.

Additionally, enhancing your flexibility through exercises like stretching and yoga can improve your range of motion and allow for a smoother and more fluid swing. Flexibility is crucial for achieving an optimal golf swing with a full shoulder turn and the ability to maintain proper spine angle throughout the swing. By regularly stretching your muscles, tendons, and ligaments, you can improve your body's flexibility and reduce the risk of muscle imbalances or restricted movements that may affect your swing mechanics. In particular, improving the flexibility of your hips, shoulders, and thoracic spine can greatly benefit your golf swing, allowing for a more efficient transfer of energy from your body to the club.

Maintaining cardiovascular fitness through activities such as brisk walking, cycling, swimming, or aerobic exercises, can improve your endurance on the course, ensuring you have the stamina to play a full round without feeling fatigued. Golf is a physically demanding activity that requires walking long distances, swinging a club repeatedly, and maintaining focus for several hours. By engaging in cardiovascular exercises, you can strengthen your heart, lungs, and circulation, enabling you to sustain your energy levels throughout a round of golf. Improved cardiovascular fitness can also enhance your recovery between shots, allowing you to maintain a consistent performance from the first tee to the final hole.

Engaging in regular exercise can also have a positive impact on your overall health, which is crucial for sustaining your golfing performance as a senior. Regular physical activity can help manage weight, control blood pressure, and reduce the risk of chronic diseases such as heart disease, diabetes, and osteoporosis. As we age, our metabolism tends to slow down, making weight management more challenging. By incorporating exercise into your routine, you can burn calories, increase your metabolism, and maintain a healthy weight.

Additionally, activities that promote weight-bearing exercises, such as walking or using resistance equipment, can help increase bone density and reduce the risk of osteoporosis, a condition where bones become weak and brittle. Exercise can also help control blood pressure, which is important for preventing cardiovascular problems that can hinder your golf game. Moreover, regular physical activity has been shown to improve insulin sensitivity, allowing for better blood sugar regulation and lowering the risk of developing diabetes. By maintaining a healthy lifestyle that includes exercise, you can reduce the likelihood of chronic diseases and enjoy an active and fulfilling golfing experience as a senior.

In addition to physical benefits, staying fit can positively impact your mental well-being as well. Exercise has been proven to enhance mood, reduce stress, and improve cognitive function. Playing golf is as much a mental game as it is physical, and maintaining mental focus and resilience on the golf course is essential. Regular exercise can help release endorphins, which are chemicals in the brain that boost mood and create a sense of wellbeing. This can contribute to a more positive state of mind, reducing anxiety, stress, and depression. Improved mental well-being can lead to increased confidence, concentration, and decision-making skills on the golf course. Moreover, exercise has been shown to improve cognitive function, including memory, attention, and concentration. By engaging in regular physical activity, you can keep your mind sharp and enhance your ability to strategize and analyse the game, allowing you to make better shots and improve your overall performance.

Additionally, engaging in fitness activities can provide social and recreational opportunities, allowing you to connect with fellow golfers and enjoy the camaraderie of the sport. Golf is inherently a social game, and participating in group exercise classes or joining golf fitness clubs can help you meet like-minded individuals and cultivate friendships. It also provides an opportunity to bond with your golfing buddies outside of the course, helping to strengthen your golfing community and making the overall experience more enjoyable. Furthermore, fitness activities can serve as a form of stress relief and relaxation, offering a break from the pressures and demands of everyday life. By dedicating time to exercise, you are prioritizing self-care and investing in your well-being, which can have a positive impact on all areas of your life, including your golf game.

It is important to note that before starting any exercise program, it is advisable to consult with your healthcare provider to ensure it is safe for you. They can provide guidance on exercise intensity, duration, and any modifications that may be necessary based on your individual needs or existing health conditions. This is especially important for seniors who may have pre-existing conditions or mobility limitations that need to be taken into consideration when designing a fitness program. Additionally, it is crucial to listen to your body and respect your limitations. Start slowly and gradually increase the intensity and duration of your exercises to avoid injuries or overexertion. Engaging in warm-up exercises and proper stretching techniques before and after your golf round can also help prevent muscle strains and injuries.

In conclusion, incorporating fitness into your routine as a senior golfer can offer a multitude of benefits. From improving your physical health and golf performance to enhancing your mental well-being and fostering social connections, staying fit can truly enhance your overall enjoyment and success on the golf course. So, embrace the benefits of fitness and swing into a healthier and more fulfilling senior golf journey.

Chapter 4: Flexibility: The Key to a Fluid Swing

Improving your golf swing requires a combination of technique, strength, and flexibility. While technique and strength are often emphasized in golf training, flexibility plays a significant role that should not be overlooked, especially for senior golfers. As our bodies age, maintaining or improving flexibility becomes increasingly important to prevent injuries and enhance performance on the course.

So, what makes flexibility essential for a fluid swing? The answer lies in understanding how the body moves through a full range of motion. When it comes to the golf swing, adequate flexibility allows your body to execute the necessary movements with proper form, posture, and balance. Without flexibility, your body may compensate by sacrificing these factors, leading to swing faults and decreased power, not to mention an increased risk of injury that comes with improper alignment and mechanics.

To improve flexibility for your golf swing, it is crucial to focus on stretching exercises that specifically target the muscles used during the swing. By incorporating a well-rounded stretching routine into your training regimen, you can develop the necessary flexibility to execute a fluid and powerful swing.

Let's dive deeper into some key stretches that can aid in increasing flexibility for the golf swing:

1. Shoulder Rotation Stretch:

The shoulder rotation stretch is an excellent exercise for golfers as it improves the range of motion in the shoulder joint, which is crucial for a smooth golf swing. To perform this stretch, stand with your feet shoulder-width apart and gently rotate your shoulders in a circular motion. Start with small circles and gradually increase the size as you feel more comfortable. This dynamic stretch warms up and loosens the muscles surrounding the shoulders and upper back, improving the range of motion in your shoulders. With increased shoulder mobility, you can achieve a more extended backswing and follow-through, allowing for a greater transfer of power to the golf ball.

2. Hamstring Stretch:

The hamstrings, located at the back of the thighs, play a vital role in maintaining proper posture and preventing lower back strain during the golf swing. Proper stretching of the hamstrings helps maintain hip stability and allows for a smoother weight shift and rotational movement in your golf swing. To perform the hamstring stretch, stand tall and place one foot on an elevated surface, such as a step or bench, while keeping your leg straight. Hinge forward at the hips, maintaining a neutral spine, and feel a gentle stretch in the back of your leg. Hold this position for about 20-30 seconds, then switch sides. Repeat 2-3 times on each leg. Regularly stretching your hamstrings will ensure that your pelvis remains stable throughout the swing, promoting a fluid and efficient movement pattern.

3. Hip Rotation Stretch:

Proper hip mobility is essential for achieving power and accuracy in your golf swing. The hip rotation stretch targets the muscles surrounding the hips and improves their mobility. To perform this stretch, sit on the ground with your legs extended in front of you. Bend your right knee and place your right foot on the outside of your left knee. Gently twist you torso to the right, using your left elbow to push against the outside of your right knee for added resistance. This seated twist stretches the muscles surrounding your hips and improves their range of motion. Optimal hip rotation allows for increased power generation and prevents excessive rotation or strain in your lower back, resulting in a more consistent and pain-free swing.

4. Torso Rotation Stretch:

The torso rotation stretch targets the muscles involved in rotating your torso during the golf swing, specifically the obliques and upper back muscles. By enhancing the flexibility of these muscles, you promote a smoother and more controlled backswing and follow-through, contributing to improved clubhead speed and accuracy. To perform this stretch, stand with your feet shoulder-width apart and clasp your hands together in front of your chest. Slowly rotate your upper body to the right, feeling the stretch in your torso and upper back. Hold this position for about 20-30 seconds, then switch sides. Repeat 2-3 times on each side. Incorporating this stretch into your routine will help maintain the necessary range of motion in your torso, allowing for a fluid and powerful golf swing.

Remember, flexibility is not something that can be achieved overnight. Engaging in a consistent and dedicated flexibility routine is the key to long-term improvement. To maximize your results, aim to perform these stretches at least three times a week, focusing on the muscles extensively used during your swing.

Always warm up before stretching by engaging in a light cardio exercise, such as brisk walking, for about five minutes. This increases blood flow to the muscles, making them more pliable and reducing the risk of injury. Throughout each stretch, remember to breathe deeply and relax into the movement, allowing for optimal stretching benefits. Incorporating a regular flexibility routine into your golf fitness regimen can significantly enhance your swing mechanics and overall performance. As you commit to your flexibility routine, you will witness increased range of motion, enhanced power, and reduced risk of injury – all of which contribute to a fluid and enjoyable golf game.

Embrace the journey towards improved flexibility, and let it unlock your potential for a more fluid and powerful golf swing that will undoubtedly leave a lasting impression on the course.

Chapter 5: Building Strength for Greater Power and Control

As we age, it becomes increasingly important to maintain and build our strength to enhance our golf game. Building strength not only improves our power on the course but also helps us maintain control and prevent injuries. In this chapter, we will explore various exercises and techniques to build strength specifically tailored for senior golfers.

Resistance Training: Resistance training, also known as strength training, involves using resistance or weights to stimulate muscle growth and improve strength. It is essential to start with lighter weights and gradually increase the intensity as your body becomes stronger and more accustomed to the exercises. Resistance training can bring numerous benefits to senior golfers, such as increased bone density, improved joint stability, enhanced muscular endurance, and reduced risk of age-related muscle loss (sarcopenia). By incorporating resistance training into your fitness routine, you can target the muscles used in your golf swing, such as the glutes, core, arms, and shoulders. Deadlifts, squats, lunges, bench presses, and bicep curls are great examples of exercises that can help build overall body strength.

Core Strength: A strong core is the foundation of a powerful golf swing. It helps stabilize your body and transfer energy efficiently from your lower body to your upper body. Poor core strength can lead to various swing faults and decrease overall performance. To strengthen your core, incorporate exercises such as planks, Russian twists, and medicine ball rotations into your fitness routine. These exercises engage the deep abdominal muscles (transverse abdominis), obliques, and lower back muscles. Additionally, practicing yoga or Pilates can significantly improve core strength and stability, as they emphasize controlled movements and balance.

Rotational Exercises: Golf is a game that heavily relies on rotational movements. Therefore, incorporating exercises that improve your rotational strength can have a significant impact on your overall performance. Rotational strength is crucial for generating power and maintaining proper sequencing throughout the golf swing. Cable wood chops, medicine ball twists, and seated medicine ball throws are all effective exercises to enhance your rotational strength and power. These exercises engage the muscles of the core, shoulders, and hips, mimicking the movement patterns of the golf swing. Incorporating exercises that challenge your rotation in multiple planes, such as diagonal cable chops and rotational lunges, can further improve your golf-specific rotational strength.

Balance and Stability: Strength alone is not enough to improve your golf game. You also need good balance and stability to maintain control throughout your swing. Balance and stability exercises help improve your body awareness and proprioception, allowing you to maintain a solid base during your swing and prevent unnecessary movements that can affect your accuracy. Single-leg squats, stability ball exercises, and balance board drills are beneficial for improving balance and stability. These exercises challenge your body to maintain stability while performing movements, thus improving muscle coordination and overall control.

Duration and Frequency: When incorporating strength training into your routine, it is crucial to consider the duration and frequency of your workouts. Aim for at least two to three resistance training sessions per week, allowing your muscles adequate time for recovery and growth. Alongside resistance training, including cardiovascular exercises, such as walking or cycling, can improve overall cardiovascular health and endurance. Additionally, flexibility exercises like stretching or yoga should be incorporated to improve joint range of motion and reduce the risk of injuries on the golf course. Remember to always consult with a fitness professional to ensure you are performing the exercises correctly and safely, and to design a customized program that suits your specific needs and goals.

Progressive Overload: To continue building strength and seeing improvements in your golf game, it is important to progressively overload your muscles. Progressive overload means gradually increasing the stress placed on your muscles over time. This can be achieved by gradually increasing the weight or resistance used, performing more repetitions, or increasing the number of sets. By consistently challenging your muscles, they will adapt and grow stronger. However, *it is important to avoid sudden increases in intensity as this can lead to injuries*. Gradual progression is key to long-term success and preventing plateaus in your strength gains.

Periodization: Incorporating a periodization approach into your strength training program can help optimize your progress and prevent overtraining. Periodization involves dividing your training program into specific phases, each with different goals and levels of intensity. These phases can include a preparatory phase, a strength-building phase, a power-building phase, and a maintenance phase. By varying the intensity and focus of your workouts throughout each phase, you can avoid burnout and keep your body challenged while preventing overuse injuries. Consulting with a fitness professional experienced in periodized training can help you design a program that aligns with your goals and maximizes your performance.

Recovery and Rest: Allowing ample time for recovery and rest is crucial when building strength. When you engage in resistance training, you create microscopic tears in your muscles, which need time to repair and grow stronger. Adequate rest between workouts and quality sleep are essential for optimal recovery. Active recovery strategies, such as foam rolling, light stretching, and mobility exercises, can also help improve circulation and alleviate muscle soreness. Remember to listen to your body and give it the rest it needs to avoid overtraining and potential injuries.

Nutrition and Hydration: Proper nutrition and hydration play a significant role in building and maintaining strength. Consuming a well-balanced diet rich in lean proteins, whole grains, fruits, and vegetables provides your body with the necessary nutrients to support muscle growth and repair. Adequate protein intake is particularly important for muscle recovery and regeneration. Hydration is also essential for optimal performance and recovery, as it helps transport nutrients to muscles and regulate body temperature. Aim to drink water consistently throughout the day and increase your fluid intake during workouts or hot weather.

By incorporating a well-rounded strength and conditioning program into your fitness routine, you can enhance your golf game, improve power and control, and reduce the risk of injuries. Starting with lighter resistance and gradually increasing the intensity will help improve your strength over time. Consistency, progressive overload, and periodization are key elements in building strength effectively. Remember to prioritize recovery, rest, nutrition, and hydration to support your strength-building efforts. With regular practice and a focus on building strength, you will notice a significant improvement in both your strength and performance on the golf course.

Chapter 6: Improving Balance and Stability on the Course

As senior golfers, maintaining balance and stability on the golf course becomes even more crucial. It can greatly impact our swing, accuracy, and overall performance. In this chapter, we will delve deeper into various exercises and techniques that will help improve your balance and stability for a stronger game.

Balance is a fundamental element in golf, as it enables us to maintain a steady stance throughout our swing. One effective exercise to improve balance is the single-leg stance. Stand on one leg and maintain your balance for as long as possible. Start with 30 seconds and gradually increase the duration as you develop stability. This exercise helps strengthen the muscles in your lower body, including your ankles, calves, and thighs, which are essential for maintaining stability during your swing.

In addition to the single-leg stance, practicing yoga can also improve your balance and stability on the golf course. Yoga poses such as the "tree pose" or "warrior pose" can strengthen your core, improve posture, and enhance overall body awareness. Regular yoga practice can also increase flexibility, which is important for a fluid swing. Furthermore, yoga helps foster a mind-body connection, which can positively impact your focus and concentration on the course.

Another aspect of balance that often goes overlooked is proprioception. Proprioception is your body's ability to sense its position and movements in space. By strengthening your proprioceptive abilities, you can improve your balance and stability on the golf course. Proprioception exercises involve challenging your body's awareness through activities such as balance boards, wobble cushions, or even performing exercises with your eyes closed. These exercises promote neuromuscular control and help refine your body's ability to make quick adjustments to maintain balance during your swing.

Stability is another element that plays a vital role in our golf game, particularly when it comes to executing powerful shots and maintaining control. One exercise that targets stability is the stability ball squat. Sit on a stability ball against a wall with your feet shoulder-width apart. Slowly lower yourself into a squat position, ensuring your knees stay in line with your toes. Hold this position for a few seconds, then return to the starting position. This exercise engages your entire lower body and core for improved stability during your swing.

Another exercise that can help improve stability is the plank. Start by getting into a push-up position and rest on your forearms, with your elbows directly below your shoulders. Engage your core, squeeze your glutes, and hold this position for as long as you can. As you strengthen your core, you will notice increased stability and control during your swing. It is important to remember that stability and balance also require adequate strength in the supporting muscles. Strength training exercises targeting the legs, hips, and core can significantly improve stability on the golf course. Exercises such as squats, lunges, deadlifts, and hip abductions will help develop strength and stability in these muscle groups. By incorporating these exercises into your regular fitness routine, you will notice improved balance, stability, and power in your swing.

Additionally, focusing on your footwork can contribute to better balance and stability on the golf course. Poor footwork can lead to swaying, shifting weight during the swing, and an overall lack of control. Ensuring you have a solid foundation starts with proper foot alignment. During your setup, align your feet slightly wider than shoulder-width apart and distribute your weight evenly across both feet. This position allows for a stable base while maintaining mobility in your lower body during the swing. Pay attention to keeping your weight cantered and avoid excessive shifting or lifting of your feet during the swing.

Furthermore, strengthening your ankle stability can greatly enhance your overall balance during the swing. Ankle stability exercises such as heel-to-toe walks, ankle circles, and calf raises can help improve the strength and control of the muscles surrounding the ankle joint. Stronger ankles provide a solid base for your swing, enabling you to maintain balance and stability throughout.

Balance and stability training should not be limited to the physical aspect alone. Mental focus and concentration play crucial roles in maintaining balance on the golf course. Incorporating mindfulness and meditation practices into your routine can help calm your mind, reduce distractions, and promote enhanced focus during your swings. When your mind is clear and focused, you can connect more deeply with your body's movements, allowing for improved coordination and balance throughout your golf game.

In conclusion, improving balance and stability is a multifaceted endeavour that involves physical exercises, mental focus, and mindful practices. Incorporating single-leg stances, yoga, proprioception exercises, footwork drills, ankle stability exercises, and mental training into your regular routine can greatly enhance your balance, stability, and overall performance on the golf course. By dedicating time and effort to these aspects of your game you will develop a stronger more confident swing and enjoy better success on the fairways.

Chapter 7: Endurance Training for Stamina and Consistency

In the game of golf, endurance is often overlooked but plays a crucial role in maintaining consistency and performance throughout 18 holes. As a senior golfer, it is essential to prioritize endurance training in your fitness routine to ensure you have the stamina to play your best game from start to finish.

Endurance training aims to improve your cardiovascular fitness, allowing you to maintain a steady energy supply to your muscles while minimizing fatigue. By developing your endurance, you can sustain a high level of performance throughout the duration of a round, leading to more consistent shots and ultimately better scores.

One of the most effective ways to enhance your endurance for golf is through cardiovascular exercises. These exercises work your heart, lungs, and circulatory system, boosting the delivery of oxygen and nutrients to your muscles. Engaging in activities such as brisk walking, jogging, cycling, and swimming not only helps to strengthen your heart and lungs but also contributes to overall weight management and reduces the risk of chronic diseases such as heart disease and diabetes.

To maximize the benefits of cardiovascular training, it is important to establish a regular routine and gradually increase the duration and intensity of your workouts. Aim for at least 150 minutes of moderate-intensity aerobic activity or 75 minutes of vigorous-intensity aerobic activity per week, spread across several days. Moderate-intensity exercise should make you feel slightly out of breath but still able to carry on a conversation, while vigorous intensity exercise should leave you feeling more breathless and unable to speak in complete sentences.

When engaging in cardiovascular exercises, it can be beneficial to monitor your heart rate to ensure you are working within your target heart rate zone. This zone is generally between 50-85% of your maximum heart rate, which can be calculated by subtracting your age from 220. By maintaining a consistent heart rate within this zone during your workouts, you can optimize your cardiovascular fitness and endurance.

In addition to traditional cardiovascular exercises, consider incorporating interval training into your routine. Interval training involves alternating between periods of high-intensity exercise and active recovery. This method not only helps improve your cardiovascular fitness but also enhances your body's ability to recover quickly, making it especially beneficial for senior golfers. For example, you could alternate between sprinting for 30 seconds and then walking or jogging for one minute, repeating this cycle for 10-15 minutes. ***However, it is important to approach interval training with caution, especially if you have any underlying health conditions or are new to vigorous exercise.*** *Start gradually and seek guidance from a fitness professional to ensure you are performing the exercises correctly and safely.*

In addition to aerobic exercises, senior golfers can benefit from incorporating resistance training into their endurance routine. Resistance training, also known as strength training, helps improve muscular strength and endurance, specifically targeting the muscles used in your golf swing. By engaging in exercises that target your core, legs, and upper body, you can develop the necessary strength to generate power and stability in your golf swing. When incorporating resistance training, start with lighter weights or resistance bands and gradually increase the load or resistance as your muscles become stronger and more conditioned. Focus on performing exercises with proper form and technique to avoid injuries and maximize effectiveness. Seek guidance from a fitness professional to design a safe and effective resistance training program tailored to your needs, taking into consideration any physical limitations or past injuries.

To further enhance your endurance and overall fitness, consider including functional exercises in your training routine. Functional exercises mimic the movement patterns commonly used in activities of daily living, including golf. These exercises engage multiple muscle groups simultaneously, improving coordination, stability, and balance. Examples of functional exercises for senior golfers include lunges, squats, planks, and medicine ball rotations.

While physical training is essential for building endurance, it is equally important to address the mental aspect of endurance. Golf is a mentally demanding sport, and developing mental fortitude can greatly contribute to your ability to endure physical fatigue on the course. Engage in activities such as mindfulness meditation, visualization, and positive self-talk to train your mind to stay focused, overcome challenges, and maintain a positive mindset during long rounds. Incorporating these mental training techniques into your routine can significantly impact your overall endurance and performance on the golf course.

In conclusion, endurance training is a critical component of a well-rounded fitness regimen for senior golfers. By improving your cardiovascular fitness, muscular endurance, and mental fortitude, you can maintain consistency and stamina throughout your golf rounds. Incorporate a variety of cardiovascular, resistance, and functional exercises into your training routine, gradually increasing intensity and duration over time. Remember to listen to your body, seek professional guidance when necessary, and stay committed to your endurance training journey. The rewards of enhanced endurance will be evident in your improved performance and enjoyment of the game of golf.

Chapter 8: Mental Focus and Resilience: Mastering the Mind-Game of Golf

As we delve deeper into the fascinating world of golf, it becomes undeniably clear that this sport is not merely a physical game, but also a deeply psychological one. The mind-game of golf holds immense power over a player's performance, and honing mental focus and resilience becomes crucial for success on the course. In this extended chapter, we will explore an array of strategies and techniques that can help senior golfers master their mental game, enhance their overall performance, and unlock their true potential.

Concentration, the ability to maintain unwavering focus throughout a round, is a fundamental aspect of the mental game in golf. However, it is not a skill that comes naturally to everyone. The mind has a tendency to drift and become easily distracted, especially amidst the tranquil green of the fairways. Senior golfers might find that their minds wander to everyday worries or dwell on past mistakes during their rounds, leading to a lack of concentration. Nonetheless, concentration can be improved through practice and deliberate effort.

One effective method to bolster concentration is through mindfulness exercises. Mindfulness involves training the mind to fully engage in the present moment, letting go of distracting thoughts and becoming fully absorbed in the task at hand. By practicing mindfulness both on and off the course, senior golfers can cultivate greater awareness and develop the ability to stay focused throughout their rounds. Techniques such as mindful breathing, body scans, and sensory awareness can help create a state of heightened concentration and enable golfers to perform at their best.

Visualization techniques also play a vital role in enhancing concentration and boosting confidence. Senior golfers can mentally rehearse shots beforehand, envisioning every detail of their desired outcome. Engaging all their senses and immersing themselves in the experience, they can effectively program their subconscious mind and prepare their body to execute the shot with precision during the actual round. Visualizing successful shots not only increases concentration but also instils a deep sense of self-belief, promoting a positive mindset and paving the way for success on the course.

Speaking of a positive mindset, it is no secret that golf can be an unpredictable and at times frustrating sport. It tests the resilience and mental fortitude of even the most experienced players. Senior golfers, with their wealth of life experiences, can tap into their wisdom to cultivate and maintain a positive attitude on the course. Optimism and resilience go hand in hand, allowing golfers to bounce back from bad shots or poor rounds with tenacity and determination. By shifting their focus away from mistakes or missed opportunities and instead concentrating on the lessons learned and the growth potential, they can maintain an unwavering positive mindset.

Managing stress and controlling emotions are essential skills in the mental game of golf. Senior golfers often face the pressure of high expectations, both from themselves and perhaps from others who expect less from them. This pressure can lead to increased stress levels on the course, which in turn can hinder performance. To effectively manage stress, it is crucial to develop relaxation techniques that can be deployed during moments of tension. Progressive muscle relaxation, deep breathing exercises, or guided imagery can help alleviate stress and promote a state of calm focus.

Equally important is emotional control. Golf has the uncanny ability to elicit a range of emotions, from frustration and anger to elation and joy. It is crucial for senior golfers to recognize and understand their emotional responses and to manage them effectively. Developing self-awareness and emotional intelligence allows golfers to maintain composure and make clear decisions, even under the most challenging circumstances. By acknowledging and accepting their emotions without letting them dictate their actions, senior golfers can maintain a sense of balance and stability on the course, leading to improved performance.

Central to mental resilience in golf is self-belief. It is the cornerstone that fuels motivation, determination, and the pursuit of improvement. As senior golfers, it is vital to trust in our abilities and have confidence in our potential, no matter our age or physical limitations. Believing in our capacity to improve and achieve our goals is the driving force that propels our growth. Cultivating self-belief involves setting realistic goals, acknowledging our progress, and celebrating our achievements along the way. It requires embracing a growth mindset, where each challenge is seen as an opportunity for learning and development. In conclusion, mastering the mind-game of golf is a lifelong endeavour, particularly for senior golfers. By developing mental focus through concentration, visualization, and mindfulness, fostering a positive mindset, managing stress and emotions with relaxation techniques, and cultivating unwavering self-belief, senior golfers can unlock their full potential on the course.

The mind is a powerful tool in the game of golf, and when harnessed effectively, it becomes the key that opens doors to improved performance, enjoyment, and fulfilment on the senior golfer's journey.

Chapter 9: Injury Prevention and Recovery: Taking Care of Yourself

As we age, prioritizing injury prevention and proper recovery techniques becomes even more crucial for maintaining our physical well-being. In this extended chapter, we will delve deeper into strategies that can help senior golfers prevent injuries on the course and recover effectively when accidents do occur.

Understanding Common Golf Injuries

To effectively prevent injuries, it is essential to have a comprehensive understanding of the most common injuries that affect senior golfers. Let's take a closer look at these conditions, along with additional information and preventive measures:

Strains: Strains occur when muscles or tendons are overstretched or torn. Senior golfers are more susceptible to strains due to age-related changes in muscle elasticity and strength. To prevent strains, it's important to engage in regular strength and flexibility training programs that target the muscle groups involved in the golf swing. Resistance training with light weights or resistance bands can help maintain muscle strength, while stretching routines that focus on the shoulders, hips, and wrists can enhance flexibility.

Sprains: Sprains occur when ligaments are stretched or torn, usually due to an awkward twist or turn. Senior golfers may be at a higher risk of sprains due to age-related changes in joint stability and balance. To prevent sprains, it's important to work on balance and stability exercises, such as standing on one leg or using a BOSU ball. These exercises can help strengthen the ankles and improve overall balance, reducing the risk of falls and subsequent sprains.

Tendonitis: Tendonitis is the inflammation of tendons due to repetitive stress or overuse. In golf, tendonitis can occur most commonly in the elbows (golfer's elbow) and wrists. Besides strengthening exercises and stretching routines, implementing proper swing mechanics and grip techniques can help alleviate excessive stress on the tendons.

Additionally, using equipment with modern shock-absorbing technologies, such as golf club grips or gloves, can help reduce vibration and stress on the tendons.

Golfer's Elbow: Golfer's elbow, or medial epicondylitis, refers to pain and inflammation on the inner side of the elbow. To prevent golfer's elbow, it's crucial to warm up properly before playing, ensuring adequate blood flow and muscle elasticity. Using proper technique during the swing, avoiding excessive gripping pressure, and taking breaks when feeling fatigued can also minimize the risk of this condition.

Back Pain: The rotational movements and torque placed on the spine during the golf swing can lead to back pain. Senior golfers might have pre-existing back issues or a decreased ability to rotate the spine, making them more susceptible to back pain. It is important to maintain good posture throughout the swing, focusing on core strength and stability exercises to support the spine. Additionally, avoiding excessive bending or twisting motions and using supportive equipment like specialized back braces or orthotic inserts can help alleviate stress on the back.

 By recognizing the early warning signs and implementing preventive measures through proper fitness routines, technique adjustments, and appropriate equipment usage, senior golfers can decrease the risk of common golf injuries.

Warm-up and Stretching

Engaging in a proper warm-up routine before hitting the golf course is essential to prepare your muscles and joints for the physical demands of the game. These additional tips for an effective warm-up can further optimize your performance and reduce the risk of injury:

Cardiovascular Warm-up: Incorporate low-impact aerobic exercises, such as jogging in place, cycling, or using an elliptical machine, to gradually increase your heart rate and warm up the muscles. This increased blood flow will enhance muscle elasticity and readiness.

Dynamic Stretching: In addition to a general warm-up, incorporate dynamic stretching exercises that mimic the motions of the golf swing. These movements should not be held statically, allowing for a continuous flow of motion, increasing joint range of motion, and warming up muscle groups effectively. Examples include arm circles, high knees, lunges with torso rotation, and leg swings.

Sports-Specific Warm-up: Once your heart rate is elevated and you have completed dynamic stretching, practice golf-specific warm-up exercises. These exercises are designed to simulate the movements and mechanics of your swing. You can start with slow practice swings with a focus on maintaining proper form and gradually increase the speed and intensity as you warm up further.

Mental Preparation: Warm-ups are not only physical but also mental. Take this time to mentally prepare for your round and focus on your strategy and goals for the day. Visualization exercises can help you imagine successful shots and build confidence.

By incorporating these warm-up strategies into your golf routine, you can optimize blood flow, improve muscle flexibility, enhance joint range of motion, and minimize the risk of muscle strains and joint injuries.

Strengthening Exercises

Strengthening exercises tailored to the needs of senior golfers can improve overall stability and reduce the risk of injury. Expanding on the previous section, here are additional considerations and exercises to enhance your strength training routine:

Core Strength: Core strength is crucial for maintaining proper posture, stability, and power generation during the golf swing. In addition to traditional exercises like planks and bridges, incorporating functional movements that mimic the rotation and weight shift during a swing can be highly beneficial. Medicine ball rotations, cable or band rotations, and pallof presses can effectively engage the core muscles.

Upper and Lower Body Strength: Full-body strength training should not be neglected. Strengthening the upper body muscles, such as the shoulders, arms, and chest, can improve the overall stability and power transfer throughout the swing. Whereas lower body exercises like squats and lunges are vital for generating power and maintaining a stable lower body base. It is important to use proper form, start with lighter weights, and gradually progress according to your abilities.

Balance and Flexibility: Maintaining or improving balance and flexibility vastly enhances swing mechanics and reduces the risk of injuries. Incorporating exercises that challenge your balance, such as single-leg stands, balance boards, or unstable surfaces like foam pads, can improve your stability in various golf positions. Alongside balance exercises, passive and active stretching routines targeting the shoulders, hips, wrists, and ankles will work to enhance flexibility necessary for a fluid swing.

When designing a strength training program, consider your fitness level, consult with a qualified fitness professional, and remember to gradually increase weights and difficulty level to avoid overexertion or potential injury.

Proper Technique and Swinging Mechanics

Working on your swinging technique is fundamental for preventing injuries. Here are additional tips to help optimize your technique and minimize the strain on your body:

Video Analysis: Utilize video analysis tools or seek the guidance of a golf instructor to analyse and refine your swing mechanics. Visual feedback can help identify areas that may be causing excessive stress or leading to poor technique. A qualified instructor can assist you in making adjustments tailored to your physical capabilities.

Tempo and Rhythm: Maintaining a smooth and consistent tempo throughout your swing can help reduce the risk of injuries. Rushed or jerky movements can put unnecessary strain on your muscles and joints. Focus on maintaining a rhythm that allows for a controlled and balanced swing.

Weight Transfer: Proper weight transfer is crucial for generating power and minimizing stress on specific joints, such as the lower back and knees. Practice drills that emphasize shifting your weight from your back foot to your front foot during the downswing, ensuring a smooth transfer of momentum. This will help prevent excessive strain on certain areas of your body.

Grip Pressure: Avoid gripping the club too tightly, as this can lead to unnecessary tension in your hands, wrists, and forearms. Maintain a relaxed grip that allows for a smooth and fluid swing. Experiment with different grip sizes or even consider using specialized grips or gloves designed to reduce vibration and stress on your hands.

Minimalistic Swing Thoughts: While it's important to be aware of your swing mechanics, overthinking can lead to tense muscles and a restricted swing. Focus on a few key swing thoughts that help you maintain proper technique and allow for a natural and smooth Movement.

Equipment and Gear Considerations

Choosing the right equipment and gear can significantly impact your golf experience and help prevent injuries. Consider these factors when making equipment decisions:

Golf Club Fitting: Ensuring that your golf clubs are properly fitted to your body's measurements and swing mechanics is crucial. An ill-fitted club can lead to compensatory movements that can strain your muscles and joints. Consult with a professional club fitter to ensure that your clubs are the right length, lie angle, and grip size for you.

Golf Shoes: Invest in a pair of golf shoes with proper support and traction. A good pair of golf shoes can improve your stability during the swing and help prevent slips and falls on the course.

Sun Protection: Protecting your skin from the sun's harmful rays is essential, especially when spending several hours on the golf course. Wear sunscreen with a high SPF, a hat or visor to shield your face, and sunglasses to protect your eyes.

Hydration: Staying properly hydrated is vital for optimal performance and recovery. Bring a water bottle with you, and make sure to drink fluids regularly throughout your round.

Recovery and Injury Management Despite preventive measures, injuries can still occur. Knowing how to effectively manage and recover from injuries is essential for staying on track with your golf goals. Here are some tips for recovery and injury management:

Immediate Treatment: If you sustain an injury on the course, it's crucial to respond promptly. Apply the PRICE method (Protection, Rest, Ice, Compression, Elevation) to reduce swelling and pain. Protect the injured area from further harm, rest and avoid putting weight on the injury, apply ice wrapped in a cloth for 20 minutes at a time, compress the area with a bandage or wrap, and elevate the injured limb if possible.

Seek Medical Attention: If the injury is severe, does not improve over time, or is accompanied by severe pain, swelling, or loss of function, it is important to seek medical attention. A healthcare professional can provide a proper diagnosis and offer guidance fo treatment and rehabilitation.

Rehabilitation: Following medical advice, engage in a structured rehabilitation program to aid in the healing process and regain strength and function. This may involve physical therapy exercises, stretching routines, or other modalities to promote healing and recovery.

Gradual Return to Golf: Once you are cleared by a healthcare professional, ease back into golfing gradually. Start with short practice sessions or light rounds of golf and gradually increase intensity and duration as your body allows. Listen to your body and avoid pushing through pain or discomfort.

Remember, it's essential to prioritize your health and well-being when it comes to golf. By taking appropriate measures to prevent injuries and engaging in proper recovery techniques, you can continue enjoying the game for years to come.

Chapter 10: Creating a Personalized Fitness Program for your Senior Golf Journey

As a senior golfer, it is essential to have a comprehensive fitness program tailored to your needs and goals. This chapter will guide you through the process of creating a personalized fitness program that will enhance your performance on the golf course while also considering your age and physical abilities.

Assess Your Current Fitness Level:

Before embarking on any fitness program, it is crucial to conduct a comprehensive assessment of your current fitness level. Take note of your strengths and weaknesses, any physical limitations, and areas of improvement. This self-assessment will help you identify the specific areas you need to focus on in your training.

Physical Fitness Assessment: Evaluate your cardiovascular fitness, strength, flexibility, balance, and endurance. This assessment can be done with the help of a fitness professional who can guide you through various exercises and tests to gauge your current physical capabilities.

Golf-Specific Assessment: In addition to a general fitness assessment, consider working with a golf pro when evaluating your golf-specific needs. They can analyse your swing, identify any physical limitations affecting your technique, and provide valuable insights to enhance your performance.

Set Realistic Goals:

Determine what you want to achieve through your fitness program. Setting realistic and achievable goals is essential to stay motivated and measure progress Consider goals such as improving clubhead speed, increasing flexibility for a fuller swing, enhancing stability for balance, or sustaining endurance and focus during a full round of golf.

SMART Goals: Set goals that are Specific, Measurable, Achievable, Relevant, and Timebound. For example, instead of stating, "I want to increase clubhead speed," a

SMART goal may be "I want to increase my clubhead speed by 5 mph within six months by following my personalized fitness program."

Seek Professional Guidance:

Consulting with a fitness professional who has experience working with senior golfers is highly recommended. They can assess your physical capabilities, create a program tailored to your needs, and provide valuable guidance throughout your journey. A fitness professional can also ensure proper form and technique during exercises, reducing the risk of injury.

Golf-Specific Fitness Professionals: Consider working with a fitness expert who specializes in golf-specific training. These professionals understand the unique demands of golf and can design exercises and programs that directly improve your game.

Warm-Up and Stretching:

Allocate time for a proper warm-up before each session or round of golf. Warm-up exercises increase blood flow to the muscles, improve flexibility and help prevent injuries. Incorporate dynamic stretches that mimic the movements of your golf swing. Focus on loosening up the major muscle groups involved in the swing, such as the shoulders, hips, and spine.

Dynamic Warm-Up: Incorporate exercises like arm circles, leg swings, torso rotations, and shoulder stretches. These movements prepare your body for the physical demands of the game and help ensure optimal performance.

Strength and Power Training:

Senior golfers can benefit significantly from strength and power training exercises. Focus on exercises that target the muscles involved in your swing, such as the core, legs, and upper body.

Resistance Training: Incorporate resistance training using weights, resistance bands, or bodyweight exercises. Examples include squats, lunges, push-ups, rows, and medicine ball slams. Resistance training improves stability, builds strength, and generates more power in your swing.

Core Strengthening: Engage in exercises that specifically target your core muscles, such as planks, Russian twists, and stability ball exercises. A strong core improves balance, helps maintain proper posture and enhances overall golf performance.

Flexibility and Mobility:

Maintaining and improving flexibility and mobility are crucial for a smooth and efficient golf swing. Incorporate exercises that target the key areas used in your swing, such as the shoulders, hips, and spine.

Stretching Routine: Develop a regular stretching routine that focuses on the major muscle groups used in the golf swing. This may include stretches for your hamstrings, hip flexors, pectorals, and shoulders. Hold each stretch for 20-30 seconds and repeat on both sides.

Yoga or Pilates: Consider adding yoga or Pilates classes to your fitness program. These practices improve flexibility, core strength, and overall body awareness, contributing to a better golf swing.

Cardiovascular Endurance:

Enhancing your cardiovascular endurance will enable you to maintain focus and stamina throughout a round of golf. Engage in cardiovascular activities that elevate your heart rate for an extended period.

Low-Impact Exercises: Activities such as brisk walking, cycling, swimming, or using an elliptical machine are excellent choices for senior golfers. Aim for at least 30 minutes of moderate-intensity cardio exercise most days of the week.

Interval Training: Consider incorporating interval training into your cardio routine. Alternating between periods of higher-intensity efforts and active recovery helps improve cardiovascular fitness while simulating the varying intensities experienced on the golf course.

Balance and Stability:

Golf requires stability and balance, particularly during your swing. Incorporate exercises that challenge your balance and proprioception, improving stability, and reducing the risk of falls.

Balance Exercises: Include exercises that require maintaining your balance, such as standing on one leg, using balance boards, or practicing tai chi or yoga poses. These exercises strengthen the muscles responsible for balance and enhance stability on the golf course.

Proprioception Training: Proprioception exercises, such as balancing on an unstable surface, can help develop the body's ability to sense its position in space. This translates to improved control and stability during your golf swing.

Recovery and Rest:

Allow ample time for rest and recovery between workouts and rounds of golf. Adequate rest helps prevent overuse injuries, allows your muscles to repair and grow stronger and ensures you can perform at your best.

Sleep and Nutrition: Prioritize quality sleep and maintain a balanced diet to support your body's recovery process. Proper nutrition provides the essential nutrients for muscle repair and growth, while sleep allows your body to rebuild and recharge.

Active Recovery: After challenging workouts or intense rounds of golf, engage in light activities like walking, swimming, or gentle stretching. This promotes blood circulation, reduces muscle soreness, and aids recovery.

Monitor Your Progress: Keep track of your progress by maintaining a log of your workouts, practice sessions, and rounds of golf. This helps you track improvements overtime and make adjustments to your fitness program as needed.

Monitoring Technology: Utilize fitness and golf-specific technology, such as fitness apps or swing analysers, to track your progress objectively. These tools provide data insights that can guide your training and highlight areas for improvement.

Remember, creating a personalized fitness program for your senior golf journey is an ongoing process. Adjustments may be needed as your needs and goals change, or as you age. The key is to listen to your body, be consistent, and enjoy the journey. Your fitness program will not only enhance your performance on the golf course but also contribute to improved overall health and well-being.

Chapter 11: Mastering the Mental Game

Golf, often regarded as a game of precision and skill, requires not only physical prowess but also mental fortitude. In this chapter, we will explore the significance of cultivating a strong mental game to enhance your performance on the golf course.

The mental aspect of golf is frequently underestimated, yet it plays an instrumental role in achieving optimal results. Golfers of all skill levels often grapple with mental hurdles like anxiety, self-doubt, and lack of concentration. By gaining mastery over the mental game, you can overcome these obstacles and elevate your overall performance on the course. One fundamental aspect of the mental game is developing mental resilience. Golf is a sport of highs and lows, and it is imperative to remain mentally strong, even amidst challenging situations. This entails cultivating the ability to stay focused, positive, and composed, enabling you to navigate through tough shots and recover from mistakes gracefully. Mental resilience is not about avoiding mistakes or obstacles but rather about bouncing back from them and using them as learning opportunities.

How can we develop mental resilience? One effective strategy is to practice mindfulness and meditation. Engaging in these practices regularly can improve your ability to stay present in the moment, maintain focus, and manage stress. By training your mind to let goof distractions and negative thoughts, you can respond to each shot with clarity and calmness. Additionally, developing a growth mindset by embracing challenges and setbacks as opportunities for growth can help build mental resilience.

Visualization is another potent tool in mastering the mental game of golf. By mentally rehearsing your shots before taking them, you can improve your focus and overall accuracy. Close your eyes and envision the ideal trajectory, distance, and feel of the shot. Allow your mind to create a vivid blueprint for success, visualizing the ball soaring through the air and landing precisely where you desire. This technique harnesses the power of imagination, instils confidence, and enhances your ability to execute shots effectively. When visualizing, it's essential to engage all your senses. Feel the club in your hands, imagine the sound of the ball striking the sweet spot, and experience the sensation of a perfectly executed swing. The more detailed and vivid your visualization, the more effectively you will be able to translate it into reality on the course. Visualization not only enhances your technical skills but also boosts self-belief, providing a mental edge to your game.

Managing your emotions is a crucial skill in mastering the mental game. Golf has a unique ability to evoke passionate emotions, both positive and negative. It is essential to control your reactions to both good and bad shots. By staying calm and composed, you can make rational decisions and avoid letting negative emotions seep into subsequent shots. Developing emotional resilience will enable you to maintain a level-headed approach throughout your round, leading to better decision-making and shot execution.

To manage your emotions effectively, it's important to cultivate self-awareness. Recognize the triggers that lead to emotional reactions on the course. Are certain shots or situations more likely to frustrate you or make you nervous? Once you identify these triggers, implement effective coping strategies, such as deep breathing or positive self-talk, to regain control. By acknowledging and understanding your emotions, you can prevent them from derailing your game.

Effective course management and decision-making are also vital components of the mental game. By strategizing and analysing the course, you can make calculated decisions that maximize your chances of success. This includes selecting the right club, planning your shots carefully, and identifying potential hazards or challenges. A proactive approach to course management reduces stress and uncertainty, providing a solid foundation for achieving consistent performance.

A helpful technique in course management is to break down the course into smaller, manageable chunks. Focus on playing one hole at a time, rather than getting overwhelmed by the entire round. Set specific goals for each hole, considering factors such as your strengths, abilities, and risk tolerance. This approach allows you to maintain focus, stay present, and adapt your strategy according to the unique demands of each hole. Confidence and a positive mindset are paramount to mastering the mental game. Believing in your abilities and maintaining an optimistic attitude significantly influence your performance on the golf course. Cultivate a growth mindset, understanding that progress and improvement are more important than perfection. Embrace the challenges that golf presents as opportunities for growth and development.

Building confidence is a multifaceted process. Firstly, develop a thorough understanding of your strengths and weaknesses as a golfer. Recognize the areas where you excel and those that require improvement. Focus on solidifying your strengths and working on your weaknesses to build a well-rounded game. Secondly, practice consistently and deliberately. The more you practice, the more confident you will feel in your abilities. Observe the progress you make over time and celebrate even the smallest accomplishments. Lastly, surround yourself with a supportive network of friends, coaches, or mentors who can provide encouragement and constructive feedback.

Furthermore, developing a pre-shot routine can greatly aid in harnessing the power of the mental game. A consistent routine, comprising specific steps and rituals leading up to a shot, prepares both the mind and body for success. It establishes a sense of familiarity, triggers focus, and enhances concentration. A pre-shot routine can include visualizing the shot, taking practice swings, deep breathing, and affirming positive thoughts.

Crafting a pre-shot routine that suits your individual style is essential. Experiment with various rituals and steps to determine what works best for you. Once established, stick to your routine consistently, regardless of the outcome of your previous shot. This consistency will create a mental anchor, helping you enter a state of focused flow and reducing any unnecessary distractions or anxieties.

In conclusion, mastering the mental game in golf is as essential as honing your physical skills. By developing mental resilience, employing visualization techniques, controlling your emotions, practicing effective course management, and fostering a positive mindset, you can elevate your overall performance on the golf course. As you integrate these mental strategies into your game, you will find yourself more focused, confident, and ready to embrace the challenges that arise. Remember, becoming a master of the mental game takes practice, consistency, and a genuine commitment to personal growth.

Chapter 12: Continuing the Journey

As a senior golfer, your journey in the world of golf is an ongoing and deeply transformative one. It is a journey that not only shapes your physical abilities but also moulds your character and reveals inner strengths you may have never known existed.

One aspect of continuing the journey involves maintaining consistent physical training, as a strong and flexible body is essential for optimal performance. Regular workouts that focus on improving your flexibility, strength, and endurance will not only enhance your game but also help prevent injuries. Incorporate exercises that target the specific muscles used in your golf swing, such as rotational exercises for your core and shoulder stability exercises. Additionally, cardiovascular exercises like walking, swimming, or cycling can improve your stamina and overall health, allowing you to tackle long rounds with ease.

However, the journey is not solely about physical prowess. It is equally important to nurture your mind and spirit. Golf is a sport that challenges you mentally and emotionally, and cultivating a strong mental game is crucial. Embrace mindfulness techniques to improve focus and concentration, as they can help you stay in the present moment and let go of distractions. Explore meditation or visualization practices to visualize successful shots and build confidence. Develop strategies to manage stress and maintain composure in high-pressure situations, as the ability to bounce back from setbacks is a defining trait of a seasoned golfer.

Furthermore, continuing the journey involves setting new goals and constantly challenging yourself. While it is essential to work on your weaknesses, also focus on harnessing and refining your strengths. Analyse your game and identify areas where you can make significant improvements. Set specific goals such as reducing your handicap by a certain number of strokes, consistently hitting longer drives, or sinking more putts from different distances. By setting clear objectives, you not only stay motivated but also have a sense of purpose in your practice sessions and rounds.

To aid in your development, seek ongoing education and guidance from experienced professionals. Working with a knowledgeable golf instructor or swing coach can help fine-tune your technique, correct any flaws, and introduce new strategies. Attend golf clinics or workshops hosted by reputable coaches or professional golfers, where you can learn from their expertise and gain valuable insights. Engaging with golf communities and forums can also provide a wealth of knowledge and tips shared by fellow golfers who have faced similar challenges and triumphs.

Additionally, remember that the journey is not just an individual pursuit. Golf is a social sport that fosters camaraderie, and the relationships formed on the course can greatly enrich your experience. Participate in golf leagues, tournaments, or charity events, where you can connect with fellow golfers and forge lasting friendships. These connections not only offer opportunities for friendly competition but also provide a support system during both the highs and lows of your golfing journey.

Moreover, truly immersing yourself in the game involves a deep understanding of its history and traditions. Dive into the rich heritage of golf by studying the great players who came before you and their techniques, strategies, and mental approaches. Explore golf literature and biographies of legendary golfers to gain insights into the nuances of the game. Understanding the evolution of golf courses, equipment, and tournament formats can also provide a deeper appreciation for the sport and its enduring allure.

Lastly, always remember to embrace the joy that golf brings. Appreciate the beauty of the courses you play, the peacefulness of the early morning tee times, and the satisfaction of a well-executed shot. Celebrate your progress, no matter how small, and find inspiration in the achievements of golfers young and old. The journey is not about reaching a destination but rather a constant evolution and self-discovery. Embrace each challenge, each new chapter, and let your love for golf drive you towards new heights of skill, fulfilment, and personal growth.

In conclusion, the journey as a senior golfer encompasses not only physical training but also mental fortitude, education, goal-setting, meaningful connections, and a deep appreciation for the history and traditions of the sport. As you continue to traverse this transformative path, remember that the journey is a never-ending one. Embrace the process with gratitude, passion, and an unwavering commitment to self-improvement.

Open your heart and mind to the great possibilities that await you, and in the vast horizon of the golfing journey, discover the depths of your true potential.

D. PATRICK

Thanks for reading! Please add a short review on Amazon and let me know what you thought!